Gabriela dos Santos Souza Barros
Alléxya A. A. Marcos
Gabriella M.G. Nogueira

Epidemiology of Ranibizumab intravitreal applications

Gabriela dos Santos Souza Barros
Alléxya A. A. Marcos
Gabriella M.G. Nogueira

Epidemiology of Ranibizumab intravitreal applications

Analysis of intravitreal applications of Ranibizumab for the visually impaired

ScienciaScripts

Imprint

Any brand names and product names mentioned in this book are subject to trademark, brand or patent protection and are trademarks or registered trademarks of their respective holders. The use of brand names, product names, common names, trade names, product descriptions etc. even without a particular marking in this work is in no way to be construed to mean that such names may be regarded as unrestricted in respect of trademark and brand protection legislation and could thus be used by anyone.

Cover image: www.ingimage.com

This book is a translation from the original published under ISBN 978-613-9-64621-0.

Publisher:
Sciencia Scripts
is a trademark of
Dodo Books Indian Ocean Ltd. and OmniScriptum S.R.L publishing group

120 High Road, East Finchley, London, N2 9ED, United Kingdom
Str. Armeneasca 28/1, office 1, Chisinau MD-2012, Republic of Moldova, Europe
Printed at: see last page
ISBN: 978-620-7-78190-4

I dedicate this work to God, for all the blessings he has given me.

Thank you

To God, for being present in my life at all times and for being the one most responsible for all the marvellous things that happen in it.

To my best friend, my husband, my constant companion. My lifelong love, who always supports me in all my choices.

To my dear parents, who are also responsible for this victory, always encouraging me throughout this journey.

To my sister, a lifelong friend, study companion and great collaborator in finalising this work.

To all my family and friends who have always believed in my choice and supported my growth. Grandparents, uncles, in-laws, sister-in-law and cousins, thank you so much.

To my patients, who always contribute to my learning, surrounding me with affection and respect.

To my friends at the counter of the Benjamin Constant Institute, who helped me a lot by picking up the medical records every day to create my database.

To my teachers who at all times contributed to my education, showing me the day-to-day of our profession.

Summary

Objectives: To evaluate the profile of intravitreal applications of Ranibizumab in a population of adults treated at the Benjamin Constant Institute in 2015, taking into account the effect on visual acuity and macular thickness after treatment. In addition, the study aims to present the main indications for this type of treatment in the aforementioned eye service.

Materials and methods: A cross-sectional study was carried out on subjects over 20 years old between March and August 2015 to analyse visual acuity and foveal thickness before and after treatment. The dose of anti-VEGF used was 0.05ml per application with a four-week interval between applications. Visual acuity measurement and post-treatment OCT were carried out around 30 days after the last application. Statistical analyses were carried out using SPSS software version 21 and the level of statistical significance was 95% with a p-value <0.05.

Results: The study showed that the main pathology related to this treatment was non-proliferative diabetic retinopathy associated with macular oedema (32.8%). After the indicated treatment with Ranibizumab, there was an improvement in mean visual acuity from 0.70 to 0.59 (logMAR) and a regression of macular thickness, seen on OCT, from 408.1 pm to 337.2 pm (p-value <0.05).

Conclusion: It can therefore be concluded that treatment with Ranibizumab in the population studied contributed to a better quality of life for the patients, as most of them showed a statistically significant improvement in visual acuity after the applications.

Keywords: Ranibizumab, macular oedema and neovascularisation.

Contents

CHAPTER 1

Introduction

The use of intravitreal anti-VEGF is increasingly routine in ophthalmological practice today, and is responsible for the treatment of numerous ocular pathologies. It basically acts by inhibiting the angiogenesis that this endothelial growth factor promotes. Studies show that VEGF-A is the factor that most induces vascular permeability and is therefore involved in the genesis of ocular neovascularisation, present in diseases such as AMD, diabetic retinopathy, vascular occlusions, among others.[1]

There are numerous drugs that are currently used to treat the aforementioned pathologies. These include Pegaptanib (Macugen[R]), which basically inhibits forms of VEGF longer than 165 amino acids. Bevacizumab, which is a humanised monoclonal antibody (Avastin[R]), acts directly against VEGF-A and all its isoforms, but its ocular use is *off-label*[2] Ranibizumab (Lucentis[R]) acts by inhibiting all isoforms of VEGF-A, and because it is a humanised antibody fragment, it easily penetrates the retina.[1] There is also Aflibercept (Eylea[R]), which is made up of the extracellular portion of the human VEGF 1 and 2 receptor associated with the Fc portion of Immunoglobulin - G1. Studies have already shown that its action is superior to other anti-VEGF drugs, with an affinity for VEGF-A 100 times greater than Ranibizumab.[3]

Although Bevacizumab is not recognised by the FDA for the treatment of ocular neovascularisation, studies show that its effect is similar to Ranibizumab, and at the end of a year both had equivalent effects in terms of improving visual acuity, being administered in the same regimen, with intervals of one month between applications.[4] New anti-angiogenic drugs are currently being tested that promise greater affinity to VEGF, such as Pazoanib, KH902 and VEGF-Trap Eye. Recent studies have shown that the latter penetrates the retinal layers up to two hundred times more than Ranibizumab.[1]

For the last thirty years, laser photocoagulation for the treatment of diabetic macular oedema has been considered the treatment of choice for this condition. However, the use of anti-VEGF has now replaced laser, as it has been shown to improve visual acuity over a longer period of time, around three years. The ETDRS compared the use of laser and Ranibizumab, showing that the latter had a favourable safety profile and good tolerance in all the studies. This was not the case with the other anti-VEGF drugs, because although they proved to be superior to laser from the point of view of better final visual acuity, studies are still limited for these other drugs.[5]

VEGF is also involved in other ocular pathologies that have choroidal neovascularisation, such as: pathological myopia, angioid striae, multifocal choroiditis, internal punctate choroidopathy, pseudoxanthoma elasticum, ocular histoplasmosis, polypoidal vasculopathy, as well as other idiopathic causes or those related to ocular trauma. However, the main ocular pathology related to this choroidal neovascularisation is AMD. -[67] There is usually no need to use higher doses than recommended for each antiangiogenic. The recommended dose, in three injections, with an interval of one month between them, is enough to improve visual acuity and reduce retinal thickness.[8] The use of 2.0mg of Ranibizumab monthly to treat polypoidal vasculopathy, for example, showed no benefit compared to the usual dose of 0.5mg, in terms of improving visual acuity and reducing subretinal haemorrhage.[9]

With the increase in life expectancy, AMD has become an important cause of reduced visual acuity in individuals over the age of 50. As a result, the use of intravitreal antiangiogenic drugs for this condition has been gaining ground in recent years. Studies such as MARINA and ANCHOR have shown a positive effect on letter gain, resulting in an improvement in final acuity maintained for up to 12 months in AMD patients treated with Lucentis.[10] It has also been shown that in cases of macular degeneration refractory to treatment with Ranibizumab, Aflibercept injection has proved to be a great alternative in these cases.[11]

Choroidal neovascularisation related to pathological myopia, although much less common than that occurring in AMD, is also worth mentioning. The use of Ranibizumab to treat this pathology also leads to an improvement in visual acuity, demonstrated by letter gain as well as a reduction in retinal thickness after treatment (RADIANCE). The use of these intravitreal antiangiogenics to treat this type of neovasclarisation has recently been approved for this purpose, and the regression of the retinal alteration can be seen during treatment with Lucentis[R] , through OCT.[12]

Several studies show the superior results of this treatment compared to laser photocoagulation, for example.[6,7,13] The literature also shows that there is no difference between the two anti-VEGF drugs currently used in ophthalmology: both Ranibizumab and Bevacizumab are equally effective in re-establishing retinal anatomy and improving visual acuity in neovascularisation resulting from pathological myopia.[13]

OVCR or ORVCR is also a very common eye condition nowadays, probably due to the large number of underlying diseases that cause this ophthalmological alteration. Studies such as CRUISE and BRAVO show that the use of Lucentis[R] to treat macular oedema related to OVCR improves not only visual acuity but also the oedema seen by OCT.[14] After diabetic retinopathy, OVCR is the second most common retinal vascular disorder, and the use of anti-VEGF drugs outperforms focal laser photocoagulation and intravitreal corticosteroid treatment. And just as in diabetic retinopathy, macular oedema is the main cause of reduced visual acuity in retinal venous occlusion[14,15]

As previously mentioned, Ranibizumab is the anti-VEGF that neutralises all isoforms of VEGF and therefore provides the fastest and most continuous improvement in visual acuity. At both 0.3mg and 0.5mg doses, Ranibizumab proved superior to placebo and laser photocoagulation in regressing macular oedema secondary to OVCR.[14]

Diabetic retinopathy is still an important cause of irreversible blindness, especially in developing countries, and diabetic macular oedema is the main cause of reduced visual acuity in these patients. Some studies suggest that the prevalence of macular oedema in patients with a recent diagnosis of diabetes ranges from 0-3%, and this figure rises with increasing years of disease.[16] The most widely used treatment for the management of diabetic macular oedema was focal/grid laser photocoagulation, but recently intravitreal anti-VEGF has been replacing it.[17]

Ranibizumab has been approved for use in all the diseases described above. Studies have shown sustained improvement in visual acuity and regression of retinal changes. The dose of Lucentis[R] recommended for intravitreal use varies from 0.3 to 0.5 mg per application. The interval between applications is 4 weeks.[18]

The retinal alteration common to the various diseases mentioned above is macular oedema, mainly secondary to diabetic retinopathy. Observation of the progression or improvement of this oedema is best monitored using OCT.

There is also neovascular glaucoma, a condition caused by an increase in intraocular pressure due to pathologies that lead to retinal ischaemia, such as venous occlusion and diabetic retinopathy, and anti-VEGF has also been approved for the treatment of this condition.[19]

More recently, a new intravitreal drug is being used to control the aforementioned diseases, known as Ozurdex[R] . This dexamethasone intravitreal implant can be used in some cases in association with Ranibizumab. A recent study showed that combining the dexamethasone implant with

Ranibizumab for the treatment of neovascularisation present in patients with AMD reduces the need for new intravitreal injections of anti-VEGF to control this pathology.[20]

Basically, these intravitreal injections are safe and don't have many side effects. The main complications described are: retinal detachment, vitreous haemorrhage, cataracts, uveitis, ocular hypertension and the most dreaded of these, infectious endophthalmitis.[21]

The occurrence of endophthalmitis varies from 1 in 1000 to 1 in 5000 cases. It has been described that the risk of endophthalmitis is higher in Bevacizumab applications compared to Ranibizumab, probably related to the moment of injection preparation, when the syringe is more exposed to bacteria, increasing the risk of infection. We emphasise that this risk is still very low, around 0.011 to 0.017%.[22]

CHAPTER 2

Objectives

To evaluate the profile of intravitreal applications of Ranibizumab in a population of adults treated at the Benjamin Constant Institute in 2015, taking into account the effect on visual acuity and macular thickness after treatment, while also emphasising the main indications for this type of treatment in the aforementioned ophthalmological service.

CHAPTER 3

Materials and methods

This cross-sectional study used as its study population adult individuals over the age of 20 with macular oedema and/or neovascularisation from various causes, seen at the Benjamin Constant Institute between March and August 2015, in the state of Rio de Janeiro. This drug was chosen because it is a safe anti-angiogenic for treating ocular diseases according to the FDA and is the most commonly used anti-VEGF in the service described.

The treatment regimen used at the Institute is based on data from the literature and is basically divided into two main groups: macular oedema (intra and sub-retinal fluid) and neovascularisation. Patients with macular oedema confirmed by fluorescein angiography and OCT of the macula followed the protocol of a monthly dose of 0.05ml (0.5mg) per intravitreal injection of Ranibizumab for three consecutive months, with a 4-week interval between applications. Patients with neovessels resulting from proliferative diabetic retinopathy or OVCR received only one dose of Ranibizumab intravitreal injection.

It is also important to emphasise that patients with choroidal neovascularisation from various causes (angioid streaks, AMD, pathological myopia), who usually had associated macular oedema, received 3 applications. No patient had both eyes treated on the same day. Some patients with RD underwent concomitant treatment with peripheral photocoagulation.

The variables studied were:
->Indication of the use of intra-vitreous antiangiogenic drugs, which took into account all patients seen in the clinic with macular oedema or retinal or choroidal neovascularisation from various causes;

- >Age of patients;

->Improvement in visual acuity after treatment: all the patients were seen before the applications, and their visual acuity was measured with the best correction, and after all the applications the visual acuity was measured again;
->Macular oedema regression on OCT: Calculated by means of the difference between the initial and final thickness of the foveal region;

The data was obtained from the institute's own file, which separates patients requiring intravitreal injections by week of application. Additional data such as: indication for treatment, number of recommended injections, gender, age, visual acuity before and after treatment were taken from the written medical records, emphasising that visual acuity after treatment was measured approximately 30 days after the last application. This acuity was measured with the patient's correction or by super pinhole. In this study, central retinal thickness was measured before and after treatment using OCT, making it easier to interpret the efficacy of the treatment when indicating a new need for photocoagulation and/or intravitreal injection. The study did not take into account angiographic data before and after treatment with Ranibizumab.

Exclusion criteria: Advanced glaucoma with the exception of neovascular glaucoma, patients with cataracts over 2+ and corneal alterations. Patients who died during the study or were lost to follow-up at any stage were also excluded.

Even patients with an indication for intravitreal ranibizumab injection without macular oedema, for example due to neovascularisation or neovascular membrane, had their OCTs assessed. Macular oedema was considered to be a central retinal thickness (foveal thickness) greater than 250 pm, measured by OCT.

Visual acuity was measured using the Snellen chart and then converted to Logmar according to the *table of notations most commonly used to represent visual acuity,* taken from the article by Messias et al. (Image 1).

Visual functions were classified according to Avila et al, BOD 2015. Mild visual impairment or no impairment was classified as normal vision and moderate to severe visual impairment was classified as low vision. These visual acuity classifications were referred to as categories throughout the study. According to the reference cited above, normal vision is classified up to 20/70 by the Snellen chart, so all values up to 20/60 (0.5 on the logMAR scale) were considered normal. Moderate to severe visual impairment included visual acuity values worse than 20/70 and better than

20/400, i.e. 20/80 to 20/320 (logMAR 0.6 to 1.2). And blindness, finally, was defined as worse than or equal to 20/400 (<1.3 on the logMAR scale), as shown in Table 1.

For the purposes of statistical analysis, all patients with a VA of less than 1.3 were classified as having a VA of 1.4 on the logMAR scale.

Analysing the variables:

The descriptive analysis used simple prevalence frequency measures, as well as measures of central tendency and dispersion (mean, standard deviation, median and quartiles). For comparative analysis, *Student*'s t-test was used for numerical variables, with a significance level of 95% (p-value < 0.05).

Statistical analyses were carried out using SPSS software version 21.

CHAPTER 4

Results

During the six months of the study, we gathered a population of 180 people, 50 per cent of whom were male and the remaining 90 female (Graph 1). The average age of the study population was 65.38 years, with a minimum age of 31 and a maximum of 92 (Table 2). Various retinal pathologies were documented in this study as indications for intravitreal therapy, the main one being PNR associated with macular oedema, followed by PDR with macular oedema, making up 32.8% and 17.8% respectively (Table 3).

We analysed 241 eyes initially in relation to visual acuity and 220 eyes in relation to OCT, emphasising that there were patients where only one eye was assessed and others with both eyes participating in the study. Finally, we ended up with 195 eyes assessed pre- and post-treatment in relation to VA and 171 eyes assessed at the initial and final moments in relation to OCT. The final figures compared to the initial ones were lower due to losses during the course of the study, such as missing information in the medical records (Table 4).

The average pre-treatment visual acuity was 0.70, rising to 0.59 post-treatment, in logMAR, with an average improvement of 0.1. With regard to OCT, the mean central retinal thickness pre-treatment was 408.1 microns, reducing to 337.2 microns, with a mean improvement of 70.87 microns. Both with a p-value < 0.05 (Table 5).

Of the patients analysed before treatment, most of them had subnormal visual function, comprising 41% of cases, followed by patients with normal vision (40% of cases) and 19% with blindness (Graph 2).

Comparing the same people before and after treatment, we had 71 people with normal vision, 84 subnormal and 40 with blindness. Of the normal patients, 95.77 per cent remained normal. Among the subnormal patients, 33.33 per cent changed to normal. And among the blind, although most continued to have this visual function, 25 per cent improved one category to subnormal vision (Table 6).

With regard to central retinal thickness, 83% of the patients analysed had pre-treatment macular oedema and 38 patients, or 17%, had central retinal thickness < 250pm (Graph 3).

Of the 26 patients who did not have oedema before the applications, 65.8% remained without macular oedema. However, with regard to the increase in central retinal thickness, of the 145 patients with macular oedema, 27.59% progressed to normalisation of central retinal thickness, and most of these patients, despite the treatment and the statistically significant improvement in macular thickness, remained with foveal thickness > 250 pm, i.e. they remained with macular oedema (Table 7).

Images 2 and 3 show a significant improvement in the central retinal thickness of the same patient with RDNP before and after treatment. The final foveal thickness was 298 microns but remained outside the normal range, confirming what was said above: despite the significant improvement in numbers, the patients still had macular oedema.

CHAPTER 5

Discussion

The results found in this study were similar to those in the literature. The disease that most required Ranibizumab therapy was diabetic retinopathy, classified by many authors as the main cause of vision loss in patients aged between 20 and 74.[23] Macular oedema is the main cause of this reduction in vision and this complication of DR is a major public health problem.[24]

The age range of the patients included in the study is compatible with that found in articles with similar objectives to this one, as suggested by Finger et al[25] , where most of the patients assessed were between 65 and 80 years old. In most of the studies, the average age varies between 60 and 70 years[2627] , as was found in this one. With regard to gender, we realise that there are wide variations in the studies. In the study by Wang et al[26] most of the patients were male. However, according to The Catt Research Group[4] , the majority of AMD patients assessed were female.

The majority of patients showed stabilisation or improvement in visual acuity after using Ranibizumab, showing that the therapy is effective in treating macular oedema and neovascularisation from the causes shown above. Studies have shown results similar to those found in this study, suggesting that improvement in VA can be sustained up to the first 4 months of follow-up.[25]

Central retinal thickness also showed regression after treatment with Ranibizumab, with macular oedema regression in most cases, maintaining a p-value <0.05. Almeida et al.[27] studied the regression of macular oedema after treatment with Ranibizumab in AMD patients in Portugal, showing improvement in macular oedema in mm^3 , with an age range of patients assessed similar to ours, as well as a predominance of women in the study, with an N much lower than the study in question and other international references. Another study of patients with AMD in China cites data very similar to that found in our study, where the average retinal thickness in microns varied from 492.44 before treatment to 476.31 after treatment.[26] confirming that therapy with lucentis at the dose used in the study outperforms placebo and ranibiizumab itself at a dose of 0.3mg.[28]

In the study, 40% of the patients who underwent intravitreal injection of Ranibizumab had normal vision, despite the indication for intravitreal therapy with Ranibizumab, and most of these patients maintained normal vision after the applications, showing that the treatment is effective in maintaining visual acuity. It may also be thought that when patients treated with Ranibizumab have normal VA, there is a greater chance of a satisfactory post-treatment result.[29] is probably due to the shorter progression time of the disease, with less damage to the retinal cells.

Data from the literature suggests that treatment with Ranibizumab can reduce the number of people with low vision and legal blindness related to diabetic MS and resulting from AMD[30] in the same way that was shown in the study in question, because even though the majority of the population studied had subnormal vision, a significant proportion of them evolved to normal vision.

Studies such as this are important for confirming the importance of intravitreal therapy today, as this treatment prevents the treated disease from progressing to greater severity and reduces the chance of retinal sequelae after treatment.[31] data found in the study only contribute to this theory by showing that most patients with the aforementioned diseases showed stabilisation or improvement of their eye disease.

Despite the study's limitations, such as a short follow-up time and therefore a small N, the results shown are compatible with those found in the literature. Even with a small population, the study responded favourably to the proposed objectives, showing statistically significant results in terms of improved visual acuity and regression of macular oedema using OCT.

Even though the study showed positive results, there were losses during the course of the study which could have been minimised if there had been better documentation of visual acuity in the medical records after the applications, thus contributing to the increase in the N. Some patients also didn't have OCT scans after the applications, limiting the number of eyes assessed and again reducing the N, making the study less significant. And the fact that we used visual acuity measured using the super pinhole in some patients who did not have their visual acuity measured after treatment may have caused some kind of error when analysing the results. Because even though we excluded patients with a higher degree of cataract, others with small crystalline opacities may have distorted the sample because they had better acuity in the super pinhole than in the refraction.

Although it was not within the scope of our study, most of the patients analysed will probably need further applications. Because even though the central retinal thickness reduced by an average of 70 microns after the applications, most of the patients after Ranibizumab therapy still had macular oedema, as shown in Table 7, suggesting the possibility of new applications to control retinal oedema.

CHAPTER 6

Conclusion

This study is relevant because it portrays the profile of patients who seek out one of the main public ophthalmology services in the state of Rio de Janeiro, and although there are similar studies in Brazil, we haven't found any scientific documentation with this profile of evaluating the most frequent demands in an ophthalmological service such as the one described, which has a large volume of patients with retinal pathologies and an approximate number of 30 intravitreal injections carried out every week.

Therefore, the study in question confirms the importance of intravitreal therapy today, because in addition to being an increasingly accessible and safe treatment, it enables sustained improvement in visual acuity and regression of the central retinal thickness, contributing to the maintenance of the usual retinal anatomy and consequently less damage to retinal cells, leading to more effective and lasting control of retinal pathology, thus contributing to a better quality of life for patients who seek our healthcare system.

CHAPTER 7

Bibliographical references

1- Garcia Filho CAA, Penha FM, Garcia CAA. Wet-amd treatment: a review in the anti-VEGF drugs. Revista Brasileira de Oftalmologia. 2012; Volume 71(1), 63-9.

2- Manna A, Oyede O, Ning B, Yang Y, Narendran N. Avastin and Lucentis: what do patients know? A prospective questionnaire survey. Journal of the Royal Society of Medicine Short Reports. 2013; 4:1-6.

3- Korobelnik JF, Kleijnen J, Lang SH, Birnie R, Leadley RM, Misso K, Worthy G, Muston D, Do DV. Systematic review and mixed treatment comparison of intravitreal aflibercept with other therapies for diabetic macular oedema (DME). BMC Ophthalmology. 2015; 15(1): 52.

4- The CATT Research Group. Ranibizumab and Bevacizumab for Neovascular Age-Related Macular Degeneration. The New England Journal of Medicine. 2011; Volume 364, N° 20.

5- Mitchell P, Wong TY. Management Paradigms for Diabetic Macular Edema. American Journal of Ophthalmology. 2014. Volume 157: 505-513.

6- Stuart A, Ford JA, Duckworth S, Jones C, Pereira A. Anti-VEGF therapies in the treatment of choroidal neovascularisation secondary to non-age-related macular degeneration: a systematic review. BMJ Open. 2015.

7- Fan C, Ji Q, Wang Y, Shu X, Xie J. Clinicai Efficacy of Intravitreal Ranibizumab in Early and Mid-Idiopathic Choroidal Neovascularisation. Journal of Ophthalmology. 2014.

8-Hikichi T. Individualised ranibizumab therapy strategies in year 3 after as-needed treatment for polypoidal choroidal vasculopathy. BMC Ophthalmology. 2015; 15:37.

9-Kokame GT. Prospective evaluation of subretinal vessel location in polypoidal choroidal vasculopathy (pcv) and response of haemorrhagic and exudative pcv to high-dose ai jiogenic therapy (an american ophthalmological society tf j. Trans Am Ophthalmol Soc. 2014; 112: 74-93.

10-Han SY, Bae JH, Oh J, Yu HG, Song SJ. Intravitreal Ranibizumab for Subfoveal Choroidal Neovascularisation from Age-Related Macular Degeneration with Combined Severe Diabetic Retinopathy. Diabetes and Metabolism Journal. 2015; 39:46-50.

11-Batioglu F, Demirel S, Õzmert E, Abdullayev A, Bilici S. Short- term outcomes of switching anti-VEGF agents in eyes with treatment-resistant wet AMD. BMC Ophthalmology. 2015; 15:40.

12-Almeida INF, Almeida LNF, Sobrinho EFA, Gomes BD, Souza GS, Rosa AAM et al. Optical coherence tomography and multifocal electroretinography of patients with advanced neovascular age-related macular degeneration before, during, and after treatment with ranibizumab. Arquivos Brasileiros de Oftalmologia. 2015; 78(2): 105-9.

13-Loutfi M, Siddiqui MRS, Dhedhi A, Kamal A. A systematic review and meta-analysis comparing intravitreal ranibizumab with bevacizumab for the treatment of myopic choroidal neovascularisation. Saudi Journal of Ophthalmology. 2015; 29:147-155.

14-Song W, Xia X. Ranibizumab for macular oedema secondary

to retinal vein occlusion: a meta-analysis of dose effects and comparison with no anti-VEGF treatment. BMC Ophthalmology. 2015; 15:31.

15-Triantafylla M, Massa HF, Dardabounis D, Gatzioufas Z, Kozobolis V, Ioannakis K, et al. Ranibizumab for the treatment of degenerative ocular conditions. Clinicai Ophthalmology. 2014.

16-Stefanini FR, Badaró E, Falabella P, Koss M, Farah ME, Maia M. Anti-VEGF for the Management of Diabetic Macular Edema. Review Article. Journal of Immunology Research. 2014.

17-Schmidt-Erfurth U, Lang G, Holz FG, Schlingemann RO, Lanzetta P, Massin P, et al. Three-Year Outcomes of Individualised Ranibizumab Treatment in Patients with Diabetic Macular Edema The RESTORE Extension Study. American Academy of Ophthalmolog. 2014; 121 (5): 1045-1053.

18-Dedania VS, Bakri SJ. Current perspectives on ranibizumab. Clinicai Ophthalmology. 2015: 9 533-542.

19-Simha A, Braganza A, Abraham L, Samuel P, Lindsley K. Anti-vascular endothelial growth factor for neovascular glaucoma. NIH Public Access Author Manuscript. 2014; 1-29.

20-Kuppermann BD, Goldstein M, Maturi RK, Pollack A, Singer M, Tufail A et al. Dexamethasone Intravitreal Implant as Adjunctive Therapy to Ranibizumab in Neovascular Age-Related Macular Degeneration: A Multicenter Randomized Controlled Trial. Ophthalmologica. 2015; 234: 40-54.

21-Rodrigues EB, Maia M, Penha FM, Dib E, Bordon AF, Júnior OM. Technique for intravitreal injection of drugs in the treatment of vitreoretinal diseases. Arquivos Brasileiros de Oftalmologia. 2008; 71(6): 902-7.

22-Sigford DK, Reddy S, Mollineaux C, Schaal S. Global reported endophthalmitis risk following intravitreal injections of anti-VE GF: a literature review and analysis. Clinicai Ophthalmology. 2015: 9 773-781.

23-Varma R, Bressler NM, Doan QV, Gleeson M, Danese M, Bower JK, et al. Prevalence of and Risk Factors for Diabetic Macular Edema in the United States. JAMA Ophthalmol. 2014; 132(11): 1334-40.

24-Stefanini FR, Badaró E, Falabella P, Koss M, Farah ME, Maia M. Anti-VEGF for the Management of Diabetic Macular Edema- Review Article. Journal of Immunology Research. 2014.

25-Finger RP, Wiedemann P, Blumhagen F, Pohl K, Holz FG. Treatment patterns, visual acuity and quality-of-life outcomes of the WAVE study - A noninterventional study of ranibizumab treatment for neovascular age-related macular degeneration in Germany. Acta Ophthalmol. 2013: 91: 540-546.

26-Wang LL, Liu WJ, Liu HY, Xu X. Singlelzlsite Baseline and Shortlzlterm Outcomes of Clinicai Characteristics and Life Quality Evaluation of Chinese Wet Age-related Macular Degeneration Patients in Routine Clinicai Practir* Chinese Medicai Journal. 2015. Volume 128 (9): 1554- 1559.

27-Almeida IN, Almeida LN, Sobrinho EF, Gomes BD, Souza GS, Rosa AA, et al. Optical coherence tomography and multifocal electroretinography of patients with advanced neovascular age- related macular degeneration before, during, and after treatment with ranibizumab. Arq Bras Oftalmol. 2015;78(2): 105-9.

28-Domalpally A, Ip MS, Ehrlich JS. Effects of Intravitreal Ranibizumab on Retinal Hard Exudate in Diabetic Macular Edema-Findings from the RIDE and RISE Phase III Clinical Trials. American Academy of Ophthalmology. 2015. Volume 122 (4):779-786.

29-Sophie R, Lu N, Campochiaro PA. Predictors of Functional and Anatomic Outcomes in Patients with Diabetic Macular Edema Treated with Ranibizumab. American Academy of Ophthalmology. 2015.

30-Varma R, Bressler NM, Doan QV, Danese M, Dolan CM, Lee A, et al. Visual Impairment and Blindness Avoided with

Ranibizumab in Hispanic and Non-Hispanic Whites with Diabetic Macular Edema in the United States. American Academy of Ophthalmology. 2015. Volume 122 (5): 982-989.

31-Ip MS, Domalpally A, Sun JK, Ehrlich JS. Long-term Effects of Therapy with Ranibizumab on Diabetic Retinopathy Severity and Baseline Risk Factors for Worsening Retinopathy. American Academy of Ophthalmology. 2015. Volume 122 (2): 367-374.

CHAPTER 8

Illustrations

Image 1: Visual acuity conversion table from Snellen (imperial) to logmar

logMAR	Angle (minute of arc)	Decimal	Imperial	Metric	Space frequency (C/°)
1,3	20,0	0,05	20/400	6/120	600
1,2	15,8	0,06	20/317	6/95	475
1,1	12,6	0,08	20/252	6/76	378
1.0	10,0	0,10	20/200	6/60	300
0-9	7.9	0,13	20/159	6/48	238
0.8	6.3	0,16	20/126	6/38	189
0,7	5,0	0,20	20/100	6/30	150
0,6	4,0	0,25	20/80	6/24	119
0,5	3,2	0,32	20/63	6/19	95
0,4	2,5	0,40	20/50	6/15	75
0.3	2,0	0,50	20/40	6/12	60
0,2	1,6	0,63	20/32	6/10	48
0.1	1,3	0,79	20/25	6/8	38
0	1,0	1,00	20/20	6/6	30
-0,1	0,8	1,26	20/16	6/5	24
-0.2	0,6	1,58	20/13	6/4	19
-0.3	0,5	2,00	20/10	6/3	15

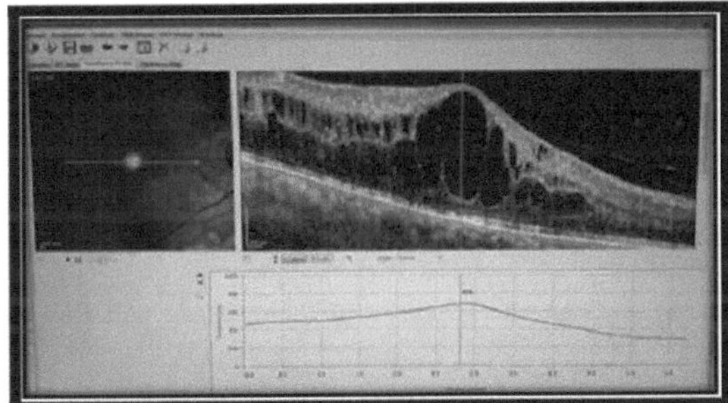

Image 2: Pre-treatment OCT of a patient with RDNP and MS

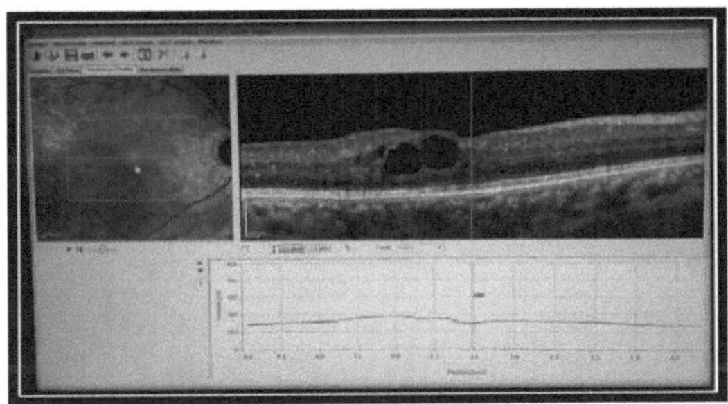

Image 3: OCT after treatment of the same patient above with RDNP and MS

Table 1: AV classification table

Visual Function	AV in logMAR
NORMAL	≤0,5
SUBNORMAL	0,6-1,2
BLINDNESS	≤1,3

Table 2: Assessment of the study population according to age

Age	
Minimum	31
Maximum	92
Average	65,38
Standard deviation	10,82

Table 3: Main diseases with indication for intravitreal therapy in the study population

Indications	N	%
RDNPcomEM	59	32,8
RDP with MS	**32**	17,8
PDR without MS	20	**11.1**
OVCR/ORVCRcomEM	20	11,1
AMD with NRVM and MS	**17**	9,4
AMD with and without NRVM	**7**	**3,9**
Cystoid macular oedema after phacactomy	5	2,8
PDR necvascular glaucoma*	**5**	2,8
Angioid striae with MNVSR to MS	5	2,8
Degenerative myopia with NRVM and MS	**2**	**1,1**
Polypoidal vasculopathy with NRVM and MS	2	**1,1**
Pseudovitiliform dystrophy with MS	**1**	0,6
MS with lamellar hole at the centre	1	0,6
Vitreous haemorrhage to be clarified	**1**	0,6
Vitelliform maculopathy with MS	1	0,6
Retinal angiomatous proliferation with MS	**1**	0,6
Chronic central serous with MS	**1**	0,6

Total		180	100,0

Table 4: Descriptive assessment of visual acuity in logMAR and central retinal thickness in microns before and after treatment with Ranibizumab

	Initial Visual Acuity	Post-Treatment Visual Acuity	Difference in visual acuity (A-P)	Initial Foveal Thickness	Foveal Thickness After Treatment	Foveal thickness difference (A-P)
N Valid	241	195	195	220	174	171
Average	0,672	0,595	0,070	403,56	336,52	70,87
Median	0,800	0,600	0,000	351,50	295,50	41,00
Standard deviation	0,445	0,478	0,358	178,42	146,97	153,77
Minimum	0,000	0,000	-1,100	153,00	148,00	-362,00
Maximum	1,400	1,400	1,200	954,00	917,00	776,00
25	0,200	0,000	0,000	262,25	233,25	0,00
50th percentile	0,800	0,600	0,000	351,50	295,50	41,00
75	1,000	1,000	0,100	522,75	408,00	115,00

Table 5: Pairwise assessment of visual acuity in logMAR and central retinal thickness in microns of patients assessed pre- and post-treatment

Peer evaluation		N	Average	Standard deviation	Peer average	Standard deviation of pairs	95% Pairwise confidence interval		p-value
							Bottom	Superior	
Acuity Visual	Top	195	0,707	0,4463	0,111	0,376	0,058	0,164	0,000
	Aftercare		0,595	0,4784					
Thickness Fbveal	Top	171	408,1	175,98	70,87	153,77	47,66	94,08	0,000
	Aftercare		337,23	148,13					

Table 6: Distribution of patients according to their visual function before and after treatment (N: 195)

Visual Acuity Classification		Initial SUBNORMAL					
		NORMAL				BLINDNESS	
		N	%	N	%	N	%
Aftercare	NORMAL	68	95,77	28	33,33	3	7,50
	SUBNORMAL	1	1,41	44	52,38	10	25,00
	BLINDNESS	2	2,82	12	14,29	27	67,50
Total		71	100	84	100	40	100

Table 7: Distribution of patients according to pre- and post-

treatment central macular thickness (N: 171)

Foveal Thickness Classification		Home			
		NORMAL		EDEMA	
		N	%	N	%
Post	NORMAL	17	65,38	40	27,59
Treatment	EDEMA	9	34,62	105	72,41
Total		26	100	145	100

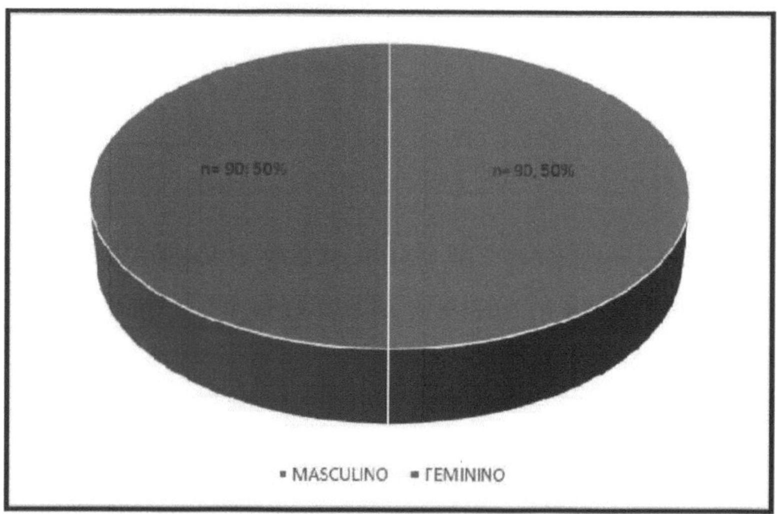

Graph 1: Number of patients by gender (180)

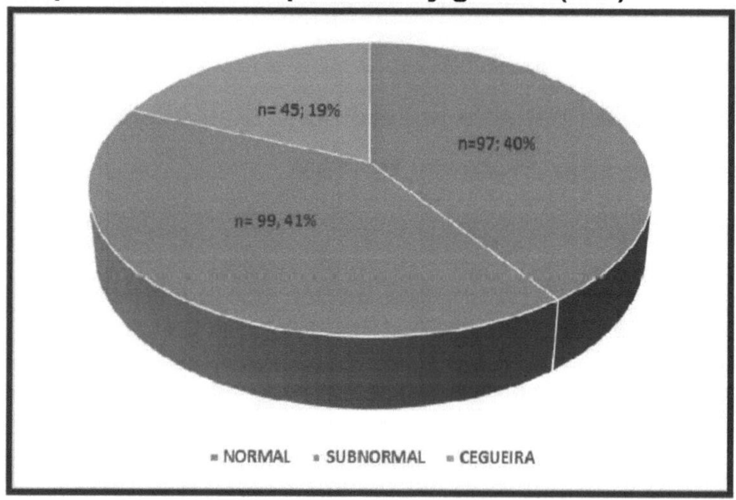

Graph 2: Categorisation of visual functions before treatment

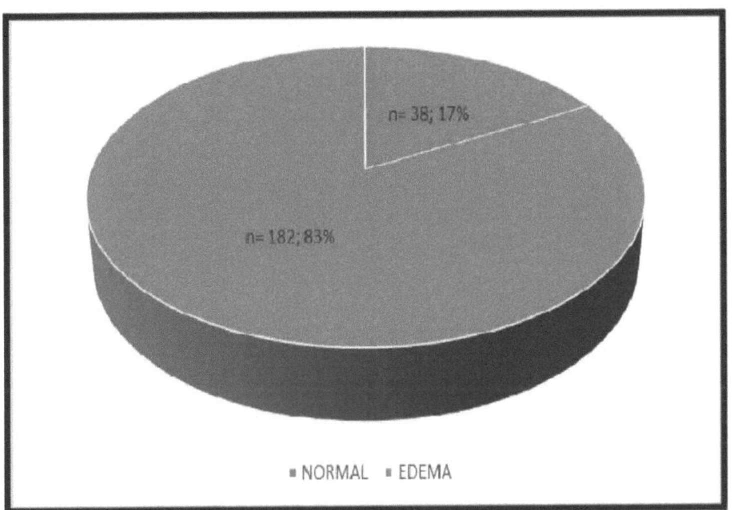

Graph 3: Classification of OCTs performed before treatment

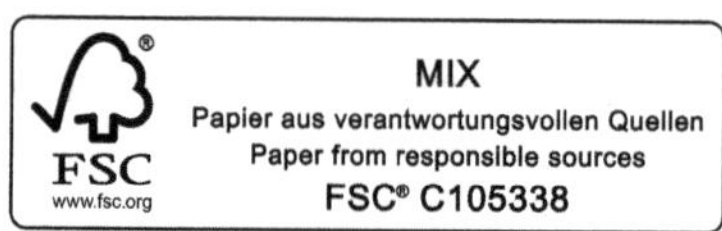

Printed by Books on Demand GmbH, Norderstedt / Germany